WHY BECAUSE

Sterling R. Stokes III

DGE PUBLISHING

Daniel Gomez Publishing

Why Because by Sterling R. Stokes III

Published by Daniel Gomez Enterprises LLC / March 2026

Publisher Contact Info: (210) 663-5954

Email: Info@DanielGomezGlobal.com

Paperback: ISBN: 978-1-970549-16-4

First Edition

Manufactured in the United States of America

DEDICATION

To the disciplined.
To the relentless.
To the ones who are done negotiating with themselves.

The time is now.

My Because…. Chloe Skye Stokes and Corinne Elizabeth Stokes!

YOU CAN-YOU WILL-YOU MUST!

TABLE OF CONTENTS

INTRODUCTION

The Most Dangerous Question in Self-Development

For the last decade, one phrase has dominated leadership conferences, self-help stages, corporate retreats, podcasts, and social media feeds:

"Find your why."

It sounds powerful.
It feels profound.
It gives people language for meaning.

But it has quietly created one of the most sophisticated forms of procrastination in modern performance culture.

We've built an entire emotional economy around inspiration.

Vision boards.
Morning affirmations.
Alignment coaching.
Purpose discovery workshops.
Identity reinvention journeys.

And yet productivity is down.
Consistency is rare.
Execution is fragile.

People are inspired more than ever…
And disciplined less than ever.

That contradiction deserves examination.

This book is not an attack on purpose.

Purpose matters.

But dependence on purpose has become a socially acceptable delay mechanism.

The world doesn't suffer from a lack of why.

It suffers from an abundance of negotiation.

And negotiation kills momentum.

If you want to change your life, your income, your body, your discipline, your standards — you don't need a deeper emotional connection.

You need inevitability.

This book will dismantle the Why illusion and replace it with something far more powerful:

The Because Method.

Not emotional ignition.

Structural certainty.

Not inspiration.

Installation.

Not clarity.

Commitment.

The time is now.

Not because you feel ready.

But because delay is expensive.

THE BECAUSE METHOD MANIFESTO

I do not move when inspired.
I move because it is required.

I do not negotiate with emotion.
Emotion negotiates with me.

I do not wait for clarity.
Clarity follows execution.

I do not revisit my purpose daily.
I execute daily.

I do not hide behind potential.
I convert potential into performance.

I do not delay.

I execute.

Because.

— Sterling R. Stokes III

CHAPTER 1

The Cult of Why — How We Were Programmed to Hesitate

There was a time when “Why” was revolutionary.

It pushed companies to think beyond profit.
It encouraged leaders to articulate mission.
It inspired individuals to seek meaning.

But like all powerful ideas, it was eventually oversimplified.

“Start With Why” became:
“Only move when you feel deeply connected.”

That shift seems subtle.

It’s not.

It changed the psychology of performance.

Because when you condition action on emotional alignment, you introduce instability.

Emotion fluctuates.

Motivation fluctuates.

Clarity fluctuates.

And anything that fluctuates cannot serve as a stable foundation for high performance.

Let's examine what actually happens when someone adopts the Why-first model.

They begin with introspection.
They search for meaning.
They explore identity.
They define a mission statement.

This process feels productive.

It creates dopamine.
It produces internal excitement.
It generates hope.

But none of it guarantees repetition.

And repetition — not inspiration — is the engine of transformation.

The human brain prefers emotion over effort.

It would rather imagine success than build it.

Purpose-searching feeds imagination.
Execution feeds discomfort.

And the brain, left unchecked, will always lean toward comfort.

This is where the trap begins.

When action feels heavy, the brain whispers:

"Maybe this isn't aligned."
"Maybe this isn't your true path."
"Maybe you need more clarity."

Notice something important.

These are not statements of fear.

They are framed as statements of self-awareness.

Which makes them socially acceptable.

Nobody criticizes you for seeking alignment.

Nobody challenges you for pausing to reflect.

But reflection, when repeated without execution, becomes elegant avoidance.

Research in behavioral psychology shows a consistent gap between intention and action. We overestimate what inspiration will produce. We assume that clarity automatically generates discipline.

It does not.

In fact, studies on implementation intentions show that behavior change increases dramatically when actions are tied to specific triggers — not emotional states.

"If it is 6AM, I train."

Not:

"If I feel motivated, I train."

The first removes negotiation.

The second invites it.

Negotiation is subtle at first.

You wake up.
You're tired.
You say, "Maybe I need rest."

You rationalize.
You justify.
You reinterpret your purpose.

And just like that, a standard dissolves.

Not because you lacked passion.

But because you left the door open.

Why leaves the door open.

Because locks it.

High performers are not superhuman.

They are structurally ruthless.

They reduce the number of decisions required to act.

They automate behavior through standards.

They don't ask daily:

"Is this meaningful?"

They declare:

"This is required."

That declaration changes everything.

Because once something becomes required, debate ends.

And performance begins where debate ends.

The Emotional Economy

Modern self-development profits from inspiration.

Motivational content spreads faster than structural discipline.

Why?

Because inspiration feels good immediately.

Structure feels heavy initially.

But heavy builds muscle.

And muscle sustains performance.

You can be deeply connected to your purpose and still lack discipline.

You can have a powerful mission statement and still procrastinate.

You can cry during a breakthrough moment and still avoid difficult tasks tomorrow.

Emotion is not evidence of execution.

Action is.

The most dangerous myth in modern performance culture is this:

“If your why is strong enough, you’ll figure out how.”

No.

If your standards are strong enough, you’ll figure out how.

Standards produce pressure.
Pressure produces adaptation.
Adaptation produces growth.

Emotion produces fluctuation.

And fluctuation destroys consistency.

The Exit Ramp Problem

Why creates exit ramps.

"I need to reconnect."
"I don't feel aligned."
"This doesn't resonate anymore."

These phrases sound evolved.

But often they mask discomfort avoidance.

Execution is boring.
Execution is repetitive.
Execution is unglamorous.

Purpose is cinematic.

And the mind prefers cinema.

But success is built in repetition — not revelation.

When you remove emotional negotiation, something shifts.

You stop asking:
"Do I feel like it?"

You start declaring:
"It gets done."

That is not cold.

That is powerful.

Because power comes from predictability.

If you cannot predict your own behavior, you cannot build momentum.

And momentum is more important than motivation.

Self-Reflection — Chapter 1

1. Where have I substituted reflection for repetition?

____

____

2. Do I revisit my purpose more than I track my performance?

____

____

3. When I stop pursuing something, do I label it misalignment instead of inconsistency?

____

____

4. What standard would change my life if it became non-negotiable?

____

____

5. If emotion were removed from my decision-making, what would I execute tomorrow?

____

____

CHAPTER 2

The Why Trap — How Purpose Becomes Permission to Stall

Let's move beyond inspiration and into mechanism.

Because the Why problem is not philosophical.

It's neurological.

When you define your actions by emotional alignment, you hand control to a fluctuating internal state.

And fluctuating states cannot produce consistent outputs.

The brain is not optimized for long-term greatness.

It is optimized for short-term safety.

That distinction matters.

When you sit down to do something difficult — build a business, write a book, train your body, make sales calls — your nervous system scans for threat.

Not physical threat.

Psychological threat.

Rejection.
Embarrassment.
Failure.
Uncertainty.

The moment discomfort appears, your brain looks for a safe interpretation.

And "misalignment" is one of the safest interpretations available.

It doesn't accuse you of weakness.

It accuses the task of incompatibility.

That subtle shift protects your identity.

This is identity-protective cognition.

Instead of admitting:
"I avoided this because it's uncomfortable."

You say:
"This isn't aligned with my purpose."

The ego stays intact.
The action disappears.

That's the Why Trap.

The Intention-Behavior Gap

Behavioral researchers have long documented what is called the intention-behavior gap.

We consistently overestimate the power of our intentions.

We say we'll train.
We say we'll start.
We say we'll build.

But intention alone produces emotional satisfaction without physical execution.

Declaring your Why creates a surge of internal meaning.

That surge feels like progress.

But feeling like progress is not progress.

This is why vision boards often stall after initial excitement.

The brain receives a reward for imagining the outcome.

And once a reward is received, urgency drops.

Why feeds imagination.

Because it feeds behavior.

Decision Fatigue and the Cost of Daily Negotiation

Roy Baumeister's research on decision fatigue reveals something critical:

Every decision consumes mental energy.

When you ask yourself every morning:
"Do I feel like training?"

You create a decision.

When you ask:
"Is this aligned with my purpose?"

You create a decision.

When you ask:
"Should I push through or rest?"

You create a decision.

By the time real strategic decisions are required, your mental bandwidth is depleted.

High performers don't have more willpower.

They have fewer daily decisions about non-negotiables.

They don't debate the gym.
They don't debate outreach.
They don't debate production quotas.

It is pre-decided.

Because it's required.

That phrase eliminates debate.

And debate is expensive.

Emotional Sophistication as Avoidance

Modern culture praises emotional awareness.

But awareness without discipline becomes indulgence.

There is a difference between understanding your emotions and obeying them.

When you constantly assess alignment, you build hypersensitivity to discomfort.

You become highly attuned to friction.

But friction is necessary for growth.

Athletes understand this.

Business builders understand this.

Elite operators understand this.

They don't interpret friction as misalignment.

They interpret friction as resistance training.

And resistance builds capacity.

Why treats friction as warning.

Because treats friction as expectation.

The Alignment Addiction

Some people are addicted to "alignment."

They chase the feeling of clarity more than the results of consistency.

They attend retreats.
They journal.
They redefine identity.
They pivot repeatedly.

But they rarely endure long enough to compound.

Compounding requires monotony.

And monotony feels uninspired.

That's the paradox.

The path to extraordinary results is boring.

It is repetition layered over time.

If you require emotional ignition to repeat, you will never compound.

And without compounding, potential remains theoretical.

The Brutal Truth

You do not need a deeper why.

You need fewer exits.

Remove the exits.

Remove the daily debate.

Remove the emotional veto power.

When something becomes required, the internal conversation changes.

It shifts from:

"Should I?"

To:

"How do I?"

That shift changes trajectory.

Because once action is assumed, strategy improves.

But as long as action is optional, strategy is irrelevant.

Self-Reflection — Chapter 2

1. Where have I labeled discomfort as misalignment?

____

____

2. What decision do I reopen every day instead of locking in?

____

____

3. If I removed emotional veto power, what would become consistent?

____

____

4. Am I more committed to protecting identity or producing results?

____

____

6. What exits must I close permanently?

____

____

Answer without ego protection.

Because clarity without honesty is useless.

CHAPTER 3

The Psychology of Because — The Language of High Earners

Now we build the alternative.

Because is not just a word.

It is a cognitive trigger.

In 1978, psychologist Ellen Langer conducted a now-famous experiment.

Participants waiting to use a copy machine were approached with different requests.

"May I use the machine?"

Compliance was moderate.

"May I use the machine because I'm in a rush?"

Compliance increased significantly.

But here's the revelation.

Even when the reason was meaningless —

"May I use the machine because I need to make copies?"

Compliance still increased.

The word “because” activated automatic processing.

The brain accepted causality.

It moved from questioning to compliance.

Now imagine applying that internally.

“I train because it’s scheduled.”

Your brain stops asking why.

It shifts to execution mode.

“I write because this is my quota.”

No debate.
No emotional scan.

Causality installed.

Cognitive Closure and Certainty

Psychological research on need for cognitive closure shows that humans prefer certainty over ambiguity.

Why introduces ambiguity.

Because introduces closure.

When you say:
“I’ll act when I feel aligned,”

You create an open loop.

When you say:
“I act because this is required,”

You close the loop.

Closed loops produce stability.

Stability produces repetition.

Repetition produces mastery.

Mastery produces results.

Grit Over Passion

Angela Duckworth's research on grit emphasizes sustained effort over time.

Not emotional intensity.

Sustained effort.

That distinction is critical.

Passion is volatile.

Grit is durable.

Because aligns with grit.

It creates repetition independent of emotional state.

High earners don't rely on inspiration cycles.

They rely on installed behaviors.

They make sales calls because that's the metric.

They train because that's the schedule.

They produce content because that's the quota.

Emotion may fluctuate.

The quota does not.

Implementation Intentions

Research by Peter Gollwitzer on implementation intentions shows dramatic increases in follow-through when actions are tied to specific triggers.

"If situation X occurs, I will perform behavior Y."

That is the structural backbone of Because.

"If it is 6AM, I train."

"If it is Monday, I review numbers."

"If it is 8PM, I write."

Not:
"If I feel motivated…"

Trigger → Action.

No debate in between.

Decision Speed and Income

High earners are not simply more intelligent.

They decide faster on pre-decided standards.

The slower you decide, the more you negotiate.

The more you negotiate, the less you execute.

The less you execute, the less you compound.

Income correlates with consistent action in revenue-generating tasks.

Not with emotional clarity.

You can deeply understand your purpose and still avoid sales calls.

But if sales calls are non-negotiable because revenue requires them, avoidance shrinks.

Because Reduces Identity Drama

When action is attached to identity, failure feels personal.

When action is attached to standard, failure feels tactical.

"I failed because I didn't follow the system."

Not:
"I failed because I'm misaligned."

That shift protects performance without protecting ego.

Because removes drama.

And drama drains energy.

The Real Advantage

Top performers don't feel less doubt.

They just don't let doubt vote.

Doubt can speak.

It cannot decide.

Because has already decided.

And once the decision is made, doubt becomes background noise.

Self-Reflection — Chapter 3

1. What daily action would increase my income if it became automatic?

____

____

2. Where do I still allow emotion to override structure?

____

____

3. What trigger can I install tomorrow?

____

____

4. What quota must become sacred?

____

____

5. If doubt lost voting power, what would change immediately?

____

____

Write one implementation intention now.

"If it is ___, I will ___."

That is your first Because installation.

CHAPTER 4

Execution Over Emotion — Installing the Because Method

You cannot outperform your standards.

You can temporarily outperform your feelings.

But you will always fall to your installed level of structure.

This is where most people misunderstand discipline.

They believe discipline is intensity.

It is not.

Discipline is architecture.

Intensity burns fast.
Architecture compounds.

The Because Method is not emotional.
It is mechanical.

And mechanics win over time.

Step 1: Remove Feelings From the Trigger

Most people use feelings as triggers.

"I feel motivated."
"I feel clear."
"I feel ready."

Feelings are unreliable signals.

They fluctuate based on sleep, stress, diet, social interaction, comparison, and environment.

If your trigger fluctuates, your output fluctuates.

Replace emotional triggers with structural triggers.

Time-based triggers.
Environment-based triggers.
Metric-based triggers.

Not:
"I write when I feel inspired."

But:
"I write from 8PM to 9PM."

Not:
"I make calls when I feel confident."

But:
"I make 25 calls before noon."

When the trigger is objective, debate disappears.

Step 2: Install Non-Negotiables

High performers operate with protected standards.

They do not protect comfort.
They protect commitments.

Choose one domain.

Health.
Revenue.
Skill.
Relationship.
Spirituality.

Choose one behavior that moves that domain forward.

Now remove negotiation.

Not:
"I'll try."

Not:
"I'll aim for."

But:
"It happens."

Because the standard requires it.

Standards are not suggestions.

They are structural boundaries.

Step 3: Eliminate Micro-Exits

Micro-exits are tiny allowances that compound into inconsistency.

"I'll skip today."
"I deserve a break."
"I'll double up tomorrow."

Each micro-exit weakens the structure.

The brain learns that pressure is temporary.

But when standards hold under discomfort, identity shifts.

You begin to see yourself as someone who executes.

Not someone who intends.

And identity built from repetition is stable.

Identity built from aspiration is fragile.

Step 4: Replace Inspiration With Metrics

Inspiration feels powerful.

Metrics are powerful.

Track:

Reps.
Revenue.
Hours.
Output.
Calls.
Meetings.
Words.
Workouts.

When performance is visible, negotiation decreases.

Ambiguity fuels avoidance.

Clarity fuels accountability.

Because what gets measured gets confronted.

Step 5: Shorten the Gap Between Decision and Action

The longer you sit between decision and execution, the more emotion re-enters.

Reduce delay.

If you decide to train, change immediately.

If you decide to call, dial immediately.

Speed protects structure.

Hesitation invites negotiation.

The Execution Equation

Standard + Trigger + Repetition = Identity Shift

Identity Shift + Time = Compound Results

Compound Results = New Reality

Notice something.

Emotion is not in the equation.

Emotion may accompany the process.

It does not drive it.

The Hard Truth

If you are inconsistent, it is not because your Why is weak.

It is because your standard is optional.

Make it non-optional. And watch what changes.

Self-Reflection — Chapter 4

1. What single non-negotiable would most improve my life?

____

____

2. Where do I allow micro-exits?

____

____

3. What metric must I track daily?

____

____

4. What trigger can replace my emotional dependency?

____

____

5. What identity would form if I repeated one action for 365 days?

____

____

Install one immediately.

Not tomorrow.

Because delay reinforces negotiation.

CHAPTER 5

Hidden Potential Dies in the Land of Why

There is a quiet tragedy happening every day.

Talented people.
Capable people.
Intelligent people.

Living beneath their potential.

Not because they lack skill.

Not because they lack intelligence.

But because they lack inevitability.

Potential is common.

Execution is rare.

And the gap between potential and performance is negotiation.

Let's examine the economics of delay.

Every day you postpone action:

Skill does not compound.
Income does not compound.
Reputation does not compound.
Confidence does not compound.

Compounding requires repetition.

Repetition requires structure.

Structure requires commitment.

And commitment requires the removal of exits.

Hidden potential is not destroyed by failure.

It is destroyed by hesitation.

Failure builds resilience.

Hesitation builds regret.

The Emotional Illusion of Readiness

You will rarely feel ready for the level you are capable of.

Readiness is built through exposure.

Not contemplation.

If you wait to feel ready before acting, you will wait forever.

Because growth requires unfamiliarity.

And unfamiliarity feels uncomfortable.

If discomfort equals misalignment in your mind, you will retreat.

But if discomfort equals expansion, you will lean in.

The interpretation changes the outcome.

Inevitability

The highest performers operate from inevitability.

They remove the question:

"Will I?"

And replace it with:

"How will I?"

That shift is transformational.

When execution becomes inevitable, results become predictable.

And predictability builds confidence.

Confidence builds speed.

Speed builds advantage.

Advantage builds wealth.

Not emotional wealth.

Tangible wealth.

Relational wealth.

Reputational wealth.

Financial wealth.

The Graveyard of Almost

The world is full of almost.

Almost started.
Almost consistent.
Almost disciplined.

Almost wealthy.
Almost fit.

Almost is comfortable.

Because almost allows identity without sacrifice.

"I'm someone who wants more."

But wanting is not doing.

And doing is the separator.

Your Fork in the Road

From this point forward, there are two paths.

Continue negotiating.

Or install inevitability.

Continue asking:
"Why should I?"

Or declare:
"Because I must."

One path feels inspiring.
The other feels demanding.

One produces temporary highs.
The other produces long-term dominance.

You do not rise to your inspiration.

You fall to your systems.

Install the system.

Because the time is now.

Not emotionally.

Structurally.

Self-Reflection — Chapter 5

1. Where in my life am I living in "almost"?

 ____

 ____

2. What opportunity is decaying because of hesitation?

 ____

 ____

3. If I made execution inevitable, what would change financially?

 ____

 ____

4. What regret would disappear in 12 months if I installed one standard today?

5. Am I more afraid of discomfort or of unrealized potential?

Sit with that last question.

Because that answer reveals your future.

CHAPTER 6

The Era of Because

Every era has a dominant belief.

There was an era of survival.
An era of information.
An era of inspiration.

Now we are entering something different.

An era of execution.

The information age gave everyone access.
The inspiration age gave everyone language.
But access and language did not create dominance.

Execution creates dominance.

The market does not reward your intentions.
It rewards your outputs.

Your family does not benefit from your potential.
It benefits from your performance.

Your body does not respond to your vision.
It responds to your repetition.

We have romanticized self-discovery.

Now we must normalize self-command.

The next level of leadership will not belong to the most inspired.

It will belong to the most inevitable.

The people who:

Wake up because it's time.
Produce because it's required.
Train because it's scheduled.
Build because they decided.

Not because they felt it.

But because they removed the option not to.

The Era of Because is not emotional.

It is structural.

And structure scales.

The Economic Shift

In a competitive economy, hesitation compounds loss.

While you reflect,
Someone else repeats.

While you realign,
Someone else builds.

While you hesitate,
Someone else compounds.

Execution is not just personal development.

It is competitive advantage.

Speed of implementation beats depth of contemplation.

Always.

The Final Divide

There are only two identities:

The Negotiator.
The Executor.

The Negotiator:
- Seeks clarity before action.
- Reopens decisions.
- Protects comfort.
- Romanticizes potential.

The Executor:
- Acts before emotion stabilizes.
- Protects standards.
- Locks decisions.
- Converts potential into assets.

Choose your identity.

Because identity shapes behavior.

And behavior shapes destiny.

Chapter 6 Self-Reflection — The Commitment Page

Write this by hand:

1. What will become non-negotiable starting today?

____

____

2. What decision will I never repoen?

____

____

3. What metric will I track daily?

____

____

4. What time based trigger will define my morning?

____

____

5. Who must I become in the next 12 months?

____

____

Then sign your name.

Not as motivation.

As contract.

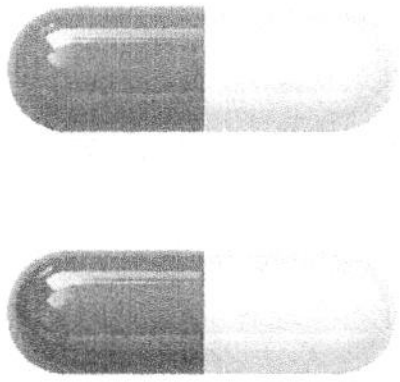

FINAL CHAPTER 7

The Death of Why. The Discipline of Because

There comes a moment in a person's life where they must choose:

Comfortable explanation
or
Uncomfortable execution.

For years, you were told to find your Why.

You were told:

• Discover your purpose.
• Clarify your passion.
• Align with your deeper meaning.
• Feel inspired.

But no one told you the dangerous truth.

Why is elastic.

Because is immovable.

Why expands.
Because contracts.

Why negotiates.
Because commands.

Why comforts identity.
Because builds results.

And the world does not reward identity.

It rewards output.

The Psychological Trap of Why

Why is seductive because it feels deep.

It feels intellectual.
It feels spiritual.
It feels aligned.

But alignment without action is fantasy.

Behavioral science has shown repeatedly:

Humans rationalize after the fact.

We do not act because we believe.
We believe because we act.

Yet Why culture reverses the equation.

It tells you:
"Once you believe enough, you will act."

No.

You act because it is required.

Belief may follow.
It may not.

Irrelevant.

Why Is the Gateway to Excuses

When your behavior is tied to Why, you unlock escape routes:

"I lost connection with my purpose."
"I'm not feeling aligned."
"This doesn't resonate anymore."
"I need clarity before I move."

All of those are emotional negotiations.

Execution does not negotiate.

Execution responds to:

Because it must be done.

Because the target requires it.

Because the standard demands it.

Because time is passing.

Because discipline is identity.

The High Earners' Secret

Top earners do not wake up inspired.

They wake up obligated.

They do not ask:
"Why am I doing this?"

They state:
"This is what gets done."

The most consistent producers in any field:

- Train at fixed hours.
- Make fixed calls.
- Track fixed metrics.
- Execute fixed systems.

They remove internal debate.

Internal debate is friction.
Friction slows output.
Slowed output kills potential.

Because eliminates debate.

Sterling's Execution Doctrine

From *Mentally Tough: Stop Delaying and EXECUTE — The Time Is Now*:

Execution is not an emotional state.
Execution is a behavioral agreement with yourself.

You do not rise to your inspiration.

You fall to your systems.

If your system requires emotion, you will be inconsistent.

If your system requires compliance, you will be inevitable.

I did not build momentum because I felt unstoppable.

I built momentum because I removed negotiation.

There were mornings I did not feel aligned.

There were seasons I questioned direction.

There were days doubt was loud.

But the system did not ask how I felt.

The system asked:

Was it completed?

That is the shift.

The Programming Cycle You Must Break

The cycle looks like this:

1. Seek purpose.
2. Feel inspired.
3. Begin strongly.
4. Lose emotion.
5. Re-evaluate Why.
6. Reset.
7. Repeat.

Years disappear inside that loop.

Because breaks the loop.

Because says:

Emotion irrelevant.
Completion required.

When you move under Because:

- You train when tired.
- You call when anxious.
- You build when uncertain.
- You execute when uninspired.

That is when identity evolves.

The Cost of Staying in Why

If you remain in Why:

You will stay talented.
You will stay intelligent.
You will stay full of potential.

You will not stay consistent.

And consistency is the only trait that compounds.

Not passion.
Not inspiration.
Not alignment.

Repetition compounds.
Precision compounds.
Relentless compliance compounds.

Why gives you relief.

Because gives you leverage.

Install the Because Protocol

Here is the irreversible shift.

Step 1: Remove emotional permission.
You do not need to feel ready.

Step 2: Define measurable outputs.
Not intentions. Not desires. Outputs.

Step 3: Time-trigger behavior.
At 6:00 AM — train.
At 9:00 AM — call.
At 1:00 PM — build.

Not when you feel like it.

When the clock says.

Step 4: Track without interpretation.
No stories.
No narratives.
Just numbers.

Step 5: Repeat without drama.

That is discipline.

That is freedom.

Freedom Is Not Emotional

Most people think freedom is doing what you want.

Wrong.

Freedom is not being controlled by how you feel.

When you can execute regardless of internal weather, you are free.

When mood no longer dictates motion, you are dangerous.

Because creates dangerous individuals.

Not aggressive.

Not reckless.

Precise.

The Identity Shift

You must decide:

Are you a person searching for meaning?

Or

Are you a person executing commitments?

One identity feels deep.

One identity builds legacy.

You cannot hold both equally.

You will drift toward one.

The Final Mirror

Look at your life right now.

Where are you inconsistent?

Where are you negotiating?

Where are you waiting for clarity?

Where are you asking Why?

Replace each with Because.

Not dramatic.
Not loud.

Quiet.
Systematic.
Daily.

That is how hidden potential becomes visible output.

The Final Commitment

Say it without emotion.

Because it must be done.

Because the standard is higher.

Because delay is over.

Because time is moving.

Because discipline is non-negotiable.

Because I execute.

Not when inspired.

Now.

Final Self-Reflection — The Irreversible Audit

1. What dream have you been protecting with explanation instead of execution?

____

____

2. Where has Why given you comfort instead of results

____

____

3. If your excuses were removed, what would your day look like?

____

____

4. What metric defines your next 30 days?

____

5. What behavior begins tomorrow without emotional consultation?

____

____

6. Who do you become if negotiation ends?

____

____

7. Are you ready to stop understanding and start executing?

____

____

EPILOGUE

The End of Negotiation

You do not need another breakthrough.

You need a boundary.

You do not need more clarity.

You need commitment.

There are only two identities:

The Negotiator.
The Executor.

Choose.

Because your life will follow your standard.

The time is now.

Structurally.

—

Sterling R. Stokes III

ENDNOTES

Sinek, Simon. *Start With Why.*
Deci, Edward & Ryan, Richard. Self-Determination Theory.
Langer, Ellen. "Mindlessness Study," 1978.
Duckworth, Angela. *Grit.*
Baumeister, Roy. Decision Fatigue research.
Gollwitzer, Peter. Implementation Intentions research.
Kahneman, Daniel. *Thinking, Fast and Slow.*

About the Author

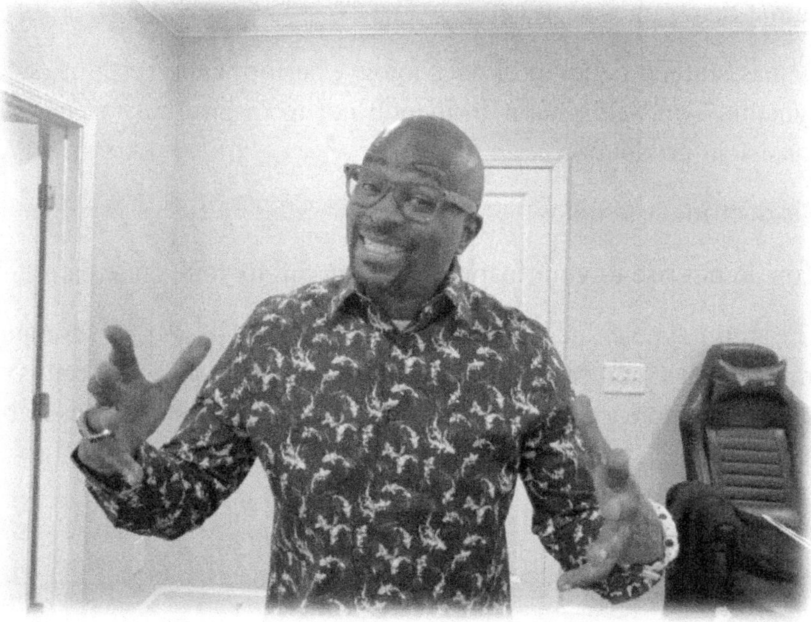

Sterling R. Stokes III is not a motivational voice.

He is an execution authority.

As the author of *Mentally Tough: Stop Delaying and EXECUTE — The Time Is Now*, Sterling has built his reputation on one core principle: performance is not emotional — it is structural.

While much of the personal development world teaches people to discover their "Why," Sterling challenges the foundation of that philosophy. His work dismantles the comfort of purpose-driven procrastination and replaces it with what he calls the Because Protocol — a measurable, disciplined system that eliminates emotional negotiation and produces results on demand.

Sterling's philosophy was not built in theory.

It was forged through real-world pressure — athletics, leadership, business execution, and high-performance environments where output determines survival.

He has studied behavioral psychology, performance systems, sales dynamics, and elite habit formation not to inspire but to engineer consistent production.

His doctrine is simple:

You do not rise to your inspiration. You fall to your systems.

Through keynote speaking, executive consulting, and performance training, Sterling equips entrepreneurs, sales leaders, executives, and competitors to remove emotional veto power, install measurable accountability, and operate with non-negotiable discipline.

He does not teach belief.

He teaches behavioral compliance.

He does not sell motivation.

He builds execution.

Sterling's message is clear:

Stop searching for meaning. Stop waiting for clarity. Stop negotiating with your potential.

Because it must be done.

And the time is now.

www.sterlingstokesIII.com

Made in the USA
Monee, IL
04 November 2026

67384105R00039